HYDROGEN

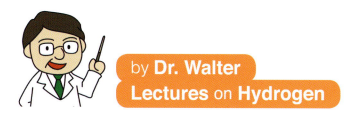

by **Dr. Walter**
Lectures on **Hydrogen**

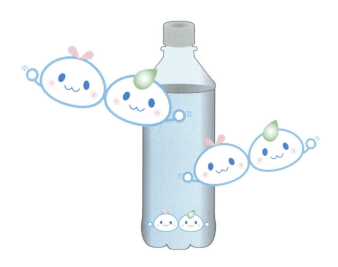

Fumiaki Ohta
Supervision : **Shigeo Ohta**

Foreword

Hydrogen is a chemical element with the chemical symbol H and atomic number 1. Two hydrogen atoms combine to form molecular hydrogen, which at standard temperature and pressure, is a colorless, odorless, tasteless, non-toxic, nonmetallic, highly combustible diatomic gas with the molecular formula H_2. Until recently, it was merely recognized as a type of inert gas.

However, in 2007, an article was published in a medical journal, proving beneficial biological activity under certain conditions. This was the beginning of hydrogen medicine, which today has proceeded successfully into its clinical trial phase.

I once read a unique article, entitled "Hydrogen-supplemented drinking water, just soda or an elixir of life?" Years later with all the scientific data, perhaps it is an "elixir of life".

Hydrogen water is well known here in Japan, and is growing in popularity in the United States and in many other countries.

In this book, I wish to clarify some common misunderstandings surrounding hydrogen and to share some results of the most recent studies.

I dream of the day when we will choose between water with H_2 gas (i.e. molecular hydrogen) or normal water with no hydrogen at meal time.

Fumiaki Ohta

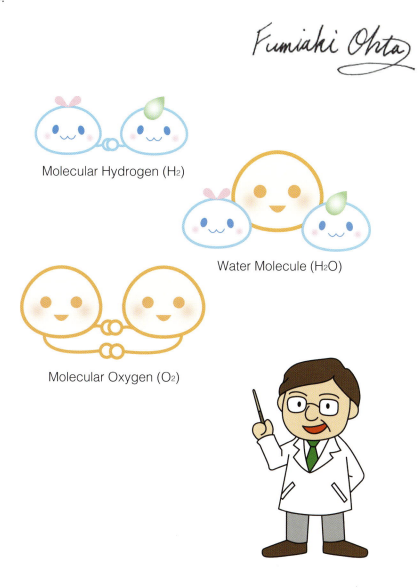

Molecular Hydrogen (H_2)

Water Molecule (H_2O)

Molecular Oxygen (O_2)

TABLE OF CONTENTS

Foreword 2

Part 1: What is hydrogen?

Hydrogen and Anti-Aging 6
Why do humans age? 8
Reactive Oxygen, the Cause of Aging 10
Good ROS and *Bad* ROS 14
Hydrogen and Vitamin C: Antioxidant Powers 16
Benefits for Brain and Reproduction! 18
How to Decrease *Bad* ROS 20
Against Oxidation, Inflammation, and Allergy 22
COLUMN Why does lifespan vary between species? 25

Part 2: Hydrogen Water, bath, and cosmetics

Hydrogen Water 26
Unit: ppm 28
COLUMN Hydrogen water and Electrolyzed water 30

Hydrogen Cosmetics	31
Controls Excessive Inflammation	32
Reducing Spots	33
Hydrogen Bath	34
Hydrogen floats around in water	35
COLUMN Can we measure hydrogen?	37
Hydrogen and Hangovers	38
Hydrogen and Genes	40
Promoting Fat Metabolism	42
Hydrogen Reducing Fatigue	43
Hydrogen does not build up	44

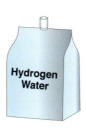
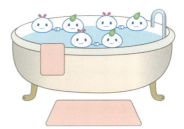

Postscript by Professor Shigeo Ohta	46
References	48
Special Thanks	50

Part 1 What is hydrogen?

Hydrogen and Anti-Aging

Hello, we are "Hydrogen"! When alone we are called "Hydrogen atoms", and holding hands, we become "Molecular Hydrogen (H_2)".

We are in a stable bond called a "Covalent Bond".
We are unstable as atoms, but stabilized in the form of Molecular Hydrogen.

stable

Some people may believe that we are highly flammable and that we easily explode near fire, this is true, but because we rapidly disperse we do not explode when added to water or inhaling the right amounts.

Hey, here comes Dr. Walter! He's an expert on Hydrogen Medicine.
Hello.

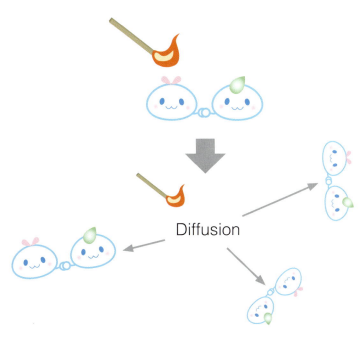

Diffusion

Hello.

Would you like to know why H_2 is beneficial to our health?

It has a lot to do with how and why we age or get sick.

Now, beginning at birth, human beings grow with time, but they will eventually start to "age".
Do you know what happens in the process of "aging"?

 Hmm, we're not sure, since we are just H, and so we don't eat or grow like you.

Part 1 What is hydrogen?

Why do humans age?

When we think in terms of energy, the definition of "being alive" means to "generate and use energy". This system of generating energy is actually where aging starts.

So where and how is energy generated?

Inside our cells, there are numerous tiny organelles called "mitochondria", where energy is generated. Let's have a closer look.

Okay! Wow, we can't see this with naked eyes.

This is a mitochondrion. It is approximately 0.001mm in diameter. They exist inside our cells, constantly multiplying, dividing, and fusing.

H_2 is much smaller than mitochondria. It is only about 1/10,000mm.

Mitochondrion is 10,000 times larger than hydrogen

Mitochondria are often illustrated in textbooks like this, but this is actually a cross-section of one mitochondrion unit. The term "Mitochondria" which we often hear is the plural form of "Mitochondrion".

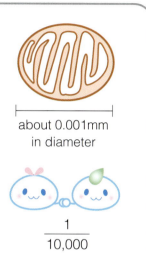

about 0.001mm in diameter

$\dfrac{1}{10{,}000}$

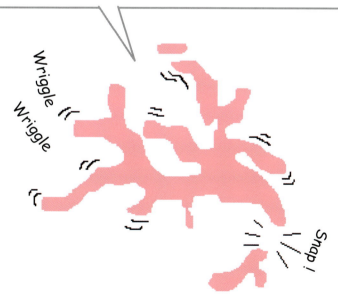

Part 1 What is hydrogen?

Reactive Oxygen, the Cause of Aging

 Mitochondria facilitate the reaction of oxygen with food to generate energy.

Sometimes, when mitochondria produce energy, electrons leak out and bond with "oxygen", which generates "Reactive Oxygen Species (ROS)".

When mitochondria become overworked they tend to produce more ROS mitochondria when they get too much stress.
Living organisms are not machines; we must continue living by repairing and reusing what have been damaged.
When there are a lot of mitochondria, they work more in sync with each other, producing less ROS, but when the number of mitochondria decrease, there are more failures in generating energy.

If you have a lot of good mitochondria, you might even look and feel younger than your actual age.

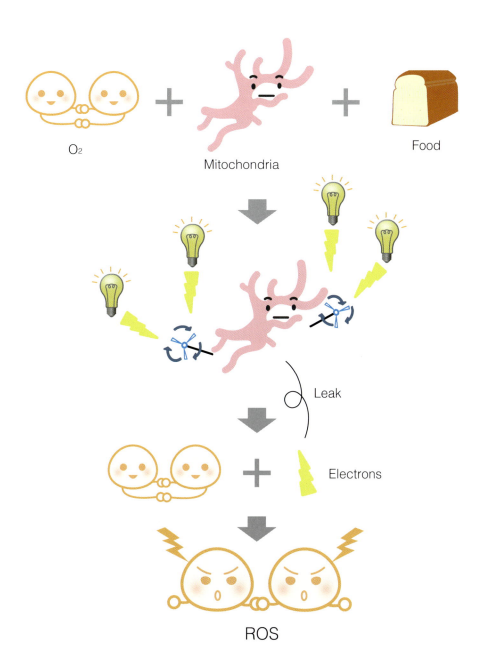

What does "Reactive" mean?

In simple words, it means a stronger tendency to combine with other molecules.

Normal O_2 can oxidize and make something rust (Oxidation Power), but the intercellular ROS generated when mitochondria are overworked have stronger oxidation effect than the normal O_2. ROS are more reactive, and will oxidize cells and proteins, meaning that they can ruin our health.

The damaged cells will be repaired, but gradually the ability to restore the cells will start to run behind, which we notice as aging or illnesses.

Hmm, so your bodies are producing energy in order to live, but this also generates ROS and can trigger the aging process. They come hand in hand...

Still, human beings are especially resistant to ROS, and so the aging process is not so fast. Plus, mitochondria also produce antioxidant enzymes that fight against ROS.

Energy-Efficient and Low Stress

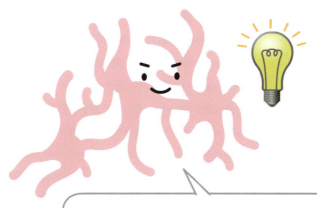

When there are many of us, we can handle requests for more energy, and we can process and supply without leaking electrons.

Less Mitochondria Cause Overwork

We produce more ROS...
We are so busy producing energy and repairing cells...
We are overloaded with too much work to do!

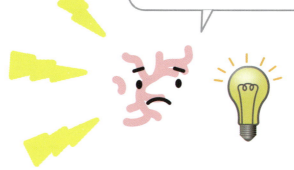

Good ROS and *Bad* ROS

 Let's talk a little bit more about ROS.

ROS are actually a general term, as there are several types of reactive oxygen species.
Some are more than 100 times stronger in oxidation power than others.
After being produced by mitochondria, ROS can continue to evolve and become stronger, and more toxic to our cells.
However, not all ROS are toxic or bad.
ROS with just the right oxidation power are actually necessary for sterilization and for the production of certain physiologically active substances. So in terms of benefits to human beings, these are regarded as good ROS.

 I see, so they can be beneficial for human health if they have the right oxidation power.

 However, even with these good ROS, overproduction can cause the repairing and processing to fall behind.

And when the mitochondria are overworked, these ROS will evolve and their oxidation power will become stronger and more toxic.

Some ROS become so strong that they oxidize everything around them. These very strong ROS can damage cells and genes, which is what turns them from good to bad to ugly for our health.

 Uh-oh, so when it's too reactive, it oxidizes everything around it...

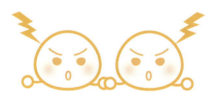

Good (Health-beneficial) ROS

Immunity, physiologically active substances, etc.
:Attacking virus with oxidation power and reducing their contagious transmission and multiplication

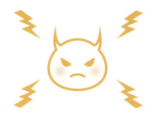

Bad (Harmful) ROS

Harms health and mitochondria by overpowering the repair process. The ROS-induced damage results in aging and illness.

Hydrogen and Vitamin C: Antioxidant Powers

👨 We researchers looked for a way to reduce aging or getting sick because of these bad ROS.
And after years of research, we found H_2.

🐰 Wow, can H_2 really do that?

👨 Yes, Before the bad ROS can do us any harm, H_2 can take care of its oxidation power, slowing our body to be oxidized. As a result of this protection from oxidation (antioxidant effect), aging and sicknesses can be reduced.

🐰 Yeah, vitamin C (and also phytochemicals, polyphenols, carotenoids, flavonoids, etc.) is most famous for its antioxidant powers, but we are in fact H_2 and have similar effects also.

👨 That's right. But in fact your antioxidant powers are fortunately not as strong as those of vitamin C.

antioxidant powers

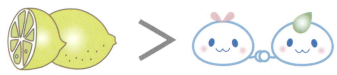

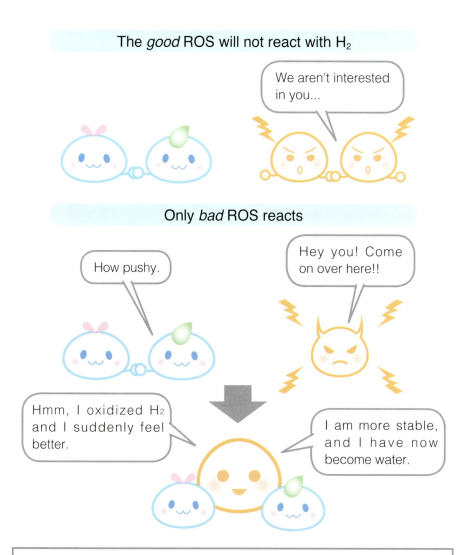

Reaction is an exchange of energy. One does not need to be strong to receive strong energy. When the receiver is strong (e. g. vitamin C), the extra energy is continually transmitted out of control. The oxidized antioxidant substances often cause further oxidation. But the mildness of H_2 makes it an ideal substance effective in taking on the excessive energy from toxic ROS and stabilizing them without getting out of control.

H_2 is oxidized by ROS in place of something else, which causes what we call the "Antioxidant" effect. H_2 is not as easily oxidized as vitamin C.

This means that H_2 reacts only with very strong and toxic ROS, and so it is more effective in protecting our health than other known antioxidant substances.

Yes, we react only with toxic ROS, which makes us great to protect your body.

Benefits for Brain and Reproduction!

H_2 reaches where it is needed due to these characteristics: dispersibility, non-polarity, and tiny size. Other drugs and compounds have difficulty reaching the required destination, at times not being delivered enough to the target part and building up where it is not needed, causing side effects because of the excessiveness.

 Important organs like brain neuron cells and reproductive organs are built to shut out foreign substances, so other antioxidant substances and drugs are unable to reach them.

Vitamin C is too big, and is only soluble to water not the cell membrane.

However, H_2 is small enough to pass through barriers and membranes, and does not leave any toxic residue. That is why, Mr. H_2, that you are effective all over our body, protecting us from the harm of bad ROS! (passing through even cartilages)

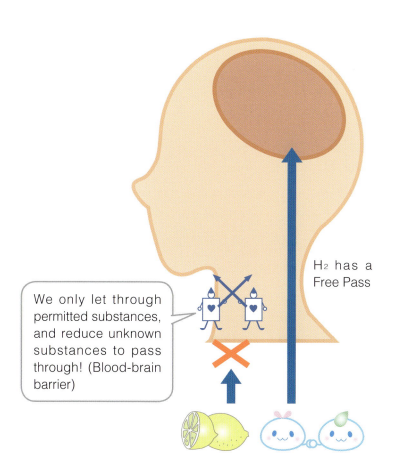

H_2 has a Free Pass

We only let through permitted substances, and reduce unknown substances to pass through! (Blood-brain barrier)

How to Decrease *Bad* ROS

 Let me give you 2 tips on how to decrease bad ROS.

● **Increasing mitochondria**

More mitochondria will improve the anti-ROS system and decrease bad ROS.
Our bodies do not produce substances in excessive quantities, and so mitochondria decrease when the body decides that we have enough energy. Therefore, by making our bodies believe that we need more energy, mitochondria will increase as a countermeasure.
For example, moderate exercise will actually produce more mitochondria. But if the workout is too light, it doesn't have much effect. Exercises that cause you slight perspiration are just the right intensity, allowing mitochondria to feel a slight energy shortage.
To create such energy shortage, you have to push yourself "slightly" more than your body is used to. Constantly repeating the same amount of workout will cause your mitochondria to get use to the intensity, so I recommend you to keep adjusting the amount of exercise for better results.

● Do not try to produce energy too quickly

Eating so fast or practicing anaerobic exercise can cause mitochondria overwork and increase ROS production. Which is okay in small amounts, but remember too much stress causes the good ROS to become bad ROS.
Consumption of alcohol, sleep deprivation, irregular living habits, and stress are all causes of ROS generation and if in excess will create the bad ROS.

A sudden energy shortage is often a result of trying to correct what is irregular. ROS overload is less likely to happen when you are calm and relaxed, but the habits like drinking and smoking are essentially toxic to our body, and the process of detoxification (from smoking and drinking) produces more ROS, which ends up being toxic.

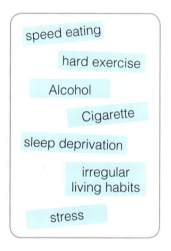

speed eating
hard exercise
Alcohol
Cigarette
sleep deprivation
irregular living habits
stress

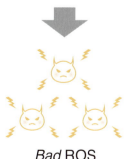

Bad ROS

Against Oxidation, Inflammation, and Allergy

🐰 I understand that H_2 can reduce the harm that bad ROS may cause.

👨 Yes, and we call this the "Antioxidant effect". But we also discovered other advantages. H_2 also has anti-inflammatory and anti-allergic effects.

Oxidation, inflammation, and allergy all used to be regarded as separate symptoms. But through observing how H_2 removes all of its causes, we have come to understand that they are closely related and in a vicious cycle. This negative cycle can cause one's health to deteriorate, so by breaking the cycle, your health can dramatically improve.
There is still a lot more studies needed, but this negative cycle probably has a genetic mechanism from too much oxidative stress.

🐰 H_2 can break the negative cycle, because it can reach and protect / influence the genes directly.

That's right. But because our senses are unique to each and every one of us, we do not all feel the effect of H_2 in the same way. The stronger you feel the effect of H_2, it may be because your original condition was caught in the vicious circle of health.

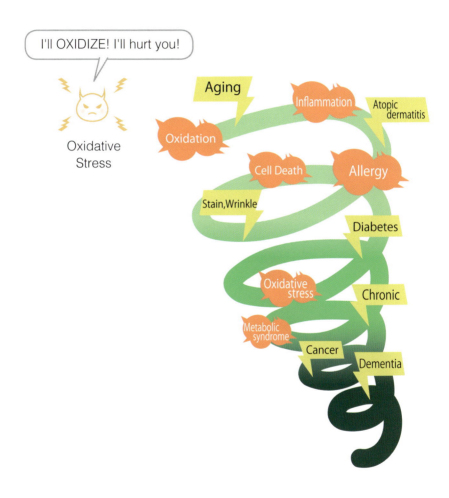

I see that H_2 can maintain your health at a very deep level.

Still, it's difficult to carry an H_2 gas container with you all day long, right?

How can you consume the adequate amount in your daily lives?

Hydrogen water is probably the simplest method. There are also hydrogen cosmetics and bath additives, so you may choose whatever fits into your lifestyle. In the future, supplements and hydrogen inhalers may become an option too.

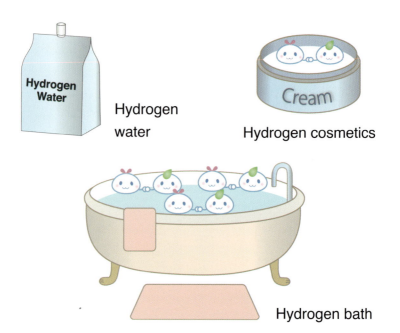

Hydrogen water

Hydrogen cosmetics

Hydrogen bath

Why does lifespan vary between species?

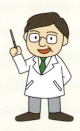

 There are so many creatures on this planet, but why do lifespans vary between species?

 One reason may be the differences in the ability of the mitochondria.
We used to believe that lifespan of creatures is in proportion to size, but human beings have a much longer lifespan than animals of similar sizes don't we? (cf. Elephants 60yrs, Lions 20yrs, Mice 2yrs)
Humans have a high ability of countering ROS and repairing damaged genes. This is why we can live longer than chimpanzees, with which we share most our genetic design. It's even presumed that the reason for our evolution is related to the fact that we can protect ourselves from ROS.

 Is it good to live a long time?

 Some may not want to live long because the longer we live, we are more likely to have unpleasant experiences, but I think we also have more opportunity to have much more fun, happy, and pleasant experiences also. Wouldn't we want to be healthy when we are experiencing such good moments? It's also important that we can pass on our knowledge to our grandchildren and great-grandchildren.

 Yes, even if you have wonderful experiences and gain valuable knowledge in your lifetime, you can't build history unless you can pass it on.

 However, our ability to protect ourselves from ROS depends largely on our living environments.
Hydrogen's anti-oxidant power against oxidation from bad ROS is a great step in the development of medicine, and towards our health and happiness.

Part 2

Hydrogen Water, bath, and cosmetics

Hydrogen Water

Hydrogen water is water infused with molecular hydrogen .
Molecular hydrogen is not "ionized" or "hydrogenated", and so the water's characteristics or its pH are unchanged.

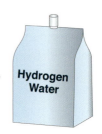

 H_2 is very tiny and easily dispersed, and so when contained in plastic bottles, H_2 leaks out and the content becomes just plain water.

 That's why aluminum containers are the most appropriate to keep us inside.

 However, even in aluminum containers, if there is hollow space inside, H_2 leaks out into the air there. So once the seal is broken, H_2 will escape.
With aluminum pouches, you can let the air out before closing them to make it last longer, which makes pouches one of the most popular packaging.

through

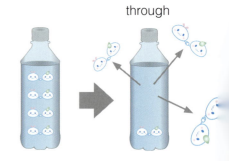

Hydrogen water seems to lose its H_2 pretty quickly once it's opened, but how fast do we have to drink it after we open it?

 Well, for example, if you pour it into a cup, it will take about 2 to 3 hours to lose about half of H_2, so you'll actually have enough time to drink it during your meal. Even if H_2 leaves, there's no change in appearance, taste or flavor, so just try to consume as much as you can before it becomes plain water.

 Is it better served cold?

 Temperature does not matter much. Just don't let it boil, as it will cause H_2 to leave. If you would like to have it warm, heat it in a water-bath before opening.

You can also make strong tea or coffee and dilute it with hydrogen water.

H_2 contained in water also has the characteristic of not being significantly affected by temperature change in terms of solubility.

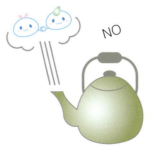 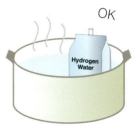

Part 2 Hydrogen Water, bath, and cosmetics

Hydrogen molecules and Hydrogen Ions

Substances with the same composition can have totally different nature depending on the bonds they have.

Let me explain the difference between " The hydrogen molecule" and "Hydrogen Ions".

With the hydrogen molecule, 2 hydrogen atoms are in covalent bonds establishing a stable state.

Hydrogen ions are often expressed as "H^+", but to be precise when they are in water, they are really: "H_3O^+".

Hydrogen ions always exist in water, and the more there are, the more acidic the water, which makes it taste sour.

In nature, bacteria produce the hydrogen molecule, but it is unlikely that natural water can contain enough molecular hydrogen from the bacteria (to be beneficial for health by drinking it).

Unit: ppm

 Let's talk numbers now.

 Do you mean the concentration of hydrogen water?

 That's right. We can usually check the amount and concentration of hydrogen products on their packages.

ORP (Oxidation-Reduction Potential) is only a reference point, so I wish we are measured more accurately. We are often described in units like ppm (parts per million), like this: "Saturation is 1.6ppm". You could use the unit mg/L instead to describe our saturation.

ppm is a ratio of mass unit, and 1.6ppm of H_2 means that the water contains about 1.6mg per liter of molecular hydrogen in the water.

If there is only about 1.6 (mg) H_2 to 1,000 (g) of water, isn't that only a tiny tiny bit?

Well, H_2 is the lightest substance, and so if we compare the weight, it seems like very little. That is probably why science textbooks write that H_2 has low solubility. In reality, if we consider the number of H_2 contained in a liter of saturated hydrogen water, $0.8mM/1000mL \times 6.02 \times 10^{23}$, we can see that we can absorb a great amount of hydrogen molecules by drinking about 300mL of hydrogen water.

That must be enough to spread throughout the body, and take care of the bad ROS.

COLUMN Hydrogen water and Electrolyzed water

 What is the difference between hydrogen water and alkaline water, or electrolyzed water?

 When we decompose water (H_2O) by electricity (Electrolysis), we get hydrogen molecules (H_2) and oxygen molecules (O_2).
Now, alkaline, from the hydroxide ions (OH^-) is when water loses just one hydrogen ($H_2O \rightarrow OH^-$). Hydrogen may be produced in the process of generating alkaline water via electrolysis.
Alkaline electrolyzed water may contain, other than H_2, a lot of alkaline (OH^-) and also metal (e. g. platinum alloy) used as electrode for the electrolysis process.

 Are alkaline water and hydrogen water the same thing?

 I prefer that they be not classified together.
You can understand that sugar water is sweet because sugar is dissolved in water, and not because adding sugar changes the taste of the water itself to become sweet, right?

 Of course! Water is water, sugar is sugar, and hydrogen is hydrogen.

 Some explain as if electrolysis changes the nature of water itself, but we need to be careful with such expressions. Some are also ignorant of the nature of hydrogen water, and incorrectly believe that even if H_2 is lost, it doesn't matter as long as the water has been electrolyzed once. We must be careful to choose hydrogen water produced by manufacturers who understand the true nature of the substance.

Hydrogen Cosmetics

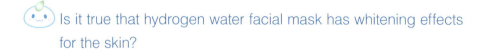 Is it true that hydrogen water facial mask has whitening effects for the skin?

Spots and marks on skin do get darker by oxidation. Results may vary, but many people have reported that their skin condition has improved with H_2.

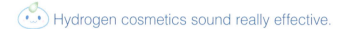 Hydrogen cosmetics sound really effective.

Through cosmetics, we can direct the effect of H_2 specifically to our skin. People have reported feeling the hydration of their skin improve, or their skin becoming firmer and younger than before by hydrogen care.

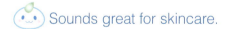 Sounds great for skincare.

There's also the anti-inflammatory effect, which might work for mosquito bites and pimples.

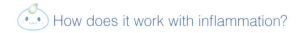 How does it work with inflammation?

Let's look into hydrogen's relationship with inflammation.

Controls Excessive Inflammation

Inflammation is a reaction of the body trying to remove an abnormal state. For example, cell damage caused by viruses, to reduce it to spread all over one's body.

Let's compare it to a wildfire. Viruses are the fire and each cell is a tree. Things would get out of control once the fire spreads all over the woods. Our body uses emergency signals called "Inflammatory Cytokines". They give the least possible sacrifice, in order to protect other healthy parts of the body.

Certain chronic conditions, for example rheumatism, are deeply related to inflammation, aren't they?

According to recent studies, we have discovered that molecular hydrogen reduces the overproduction of inflammatory cytokines. We also recently found out that when molecular hydrogen protects cells from ROS oxidation(free radical chain reaction), it actually modifies the cell membranes and regulates gene expression. You can learn more about this exciting discovery made in 2016 from the paper cited on page48-49!

So H_2 decreases unnecessary cytokines without overdoing it.

Reducing Spots

 H_2 is also efficient against ultraviolet rays.

UV exposure generates vitamin D and strengthens our immune system, but can also cause spots and freckles.

 That's why you need sunscreen.

 Sunscreens protect our skin by their UV reflective component, but they can also generate ROS. This may be what makes us feel that certain sunscreens stress our skin.

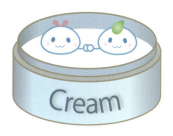

 Can H_2 improve the situation?

 Yes. Our skin is damaged by oxidation, but consuming food containing antioxidants (fruits and vegetables with vitamins, polyphenols, carotenoids, flavonoids, etc.) can help keep clear and give a healthy complexion. H_2 is definitely effective in maintaining our beauty.

Hydrogen Bath

 Is bathing in hydrogen water different from drinking it?

 By bathing in it, H_2 can seep in through our skin, and in about 10 minutes will have reached the cells all over our body, in about the same amount of time as does drinking hydrogen water. It may be difficult to fill a bathtub with hydrogen water, so there are "Hydrogen-generating bath additives (H_2 bath powder)".

 So you can ingest H_2 from within by drinking the water, and from outside by bathing in it.

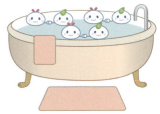

 That's right, I especially recommend hydrogen bath to those who can't drink very much water.
Molecular Hydrogen also suppresses excessive lactate (lactic acid), so it's perfect for fatigue. Also hydrogen bath promotes blood circulation and perspiration, so it works for muscle fatigue too.
In order to reduce aging and illness, it's important to improve our daily lifestyle. By being careful to "lead a lifestyle that decreases Bad ROS production" and "properly process Bad ROS" once it has been produced, you will be able to lead a healthy life for sure.

Hydrogen floats around in water

 What are H_2 like in hydrogen water and hydrogen bath?

 Molecular Hydrogen is infused into the water as it is.
Imagine molecular oxygen (O_2). Humans breath air and extract the O_2 floating around in the air. Fishes breath in the water and extract the O_2 diffused in the water. They are both the same O_2. Likewise, H_2 inside hydrogen water and hydrogen bath are both the same thing, just H_2 (hydrogen gas).

 Is it more effective to inhale hydrogen gas than to drink hydrogen water?

 I wouldn't say so. From recent research, we know that inhaling hydrogen is effective in a concentration of over 1%, which will result in reaching the organ at about 20μg/L.
By drinking hydrogen water produced under reliable quality control, roughly the same amount of H_2 will reach our organs.

 In that case, drinking hydrogen water everyday sounds so much easier than inhaling gas!

Do you know the difference between "Hydrogen Concentration" and "Oxidation-Reduction Potential (ORP)"?

Hydrogen concentration is the amount of hydrogen in the water, right? What does Oxidation-Reduction Potential measure?

ORP (measured in millivolts [mV]) signifies the "oxidation status" within liquid solution. For example, oxygen has oxidative power so if there are a lot of oxygen in the water, its ORP will be +mV (positive millivolt).

Hydrogen has reducing power, so hydrogen water will be -mV (negative millivolt). This is based on the Nernst equation and is value of the ratio given by the total reducing species (e. g. H_2) over the total oxidizing species (e. g. O_2, HOCl, etc.).

So ORP value doesn't show how much hydrogen it contains?

That's right. It is just a ratio, which is why alkaline water will also come out as -mV (Low H^+ ions and high OH^- ions), but it doesn't indicate actual antioxidant effects.
Reduction (antioxidant) and alkaline are not the same thing.

So we must watch out, because hydrogen water has negative ORP but not all liquids with negative ORP are hydrogen water!

Can we measure hydrogen?

 H_2 is transparent, tasteless and odorless, so can we measure its amount?

 Of course, we can. It would be impossible to study something without being able to measure it. There are machines that can measure molecular hydrogen by methods like gas chromatography and specially designed electrodes.
"Science" consists of "reproducibility" and "quantitatively" after all.

 It's a proven fact that H_2 has antioxidant effects within animal bodies, and the amount of hydrogen that dissolves in water is determined by the condition (e. g. temperature and pressure).

 Yes, some people seem to question the extraordinary effects of hydrogen, but they are all based on scientific grounds.

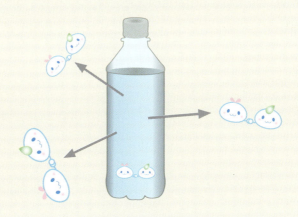

Hydrogen and Hangovers

🧑 Mmm, this wine is delicious... I shouldn't have too much though, or I'll get hung-over.

💧 Don't drink too much. It's bad for your health.

🧑 But moderate amount of alcohol promotes blood circulation, and having fun is a great way to relieve stress.

💧 Still, hangovers are harmful!

🧑 You're right, the process of decomposing alcohol is similar to how we fight against ROS. We all have different alcohol tolerances, and once we exceed our limit, it causes ROS overproduction. This can lead to hangover sicknesses and headaches.

💧 That's why H_2 is effective to hangovers.

🧑 You can even have your whiskey with hydrogen water!

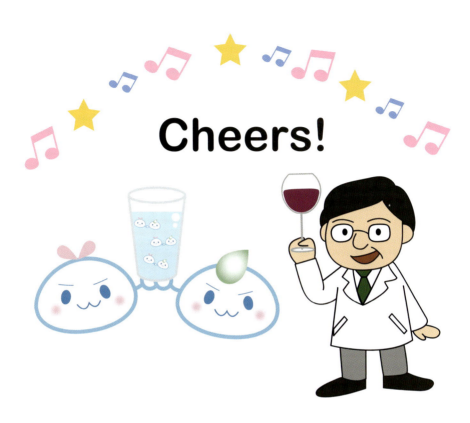

Potential for Agriculture

Plants have mitochondria too, there have been attempts to effectively employ H_2 in agriculture. H_2 can help plants fight against salt damages, and promote better growth, quality and lasting freshness.

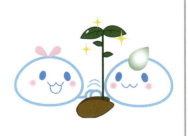

Hydrogen and Genes

 Now let's talk about some of the latest discoveries about the relationship between H_2 and our genes.

 What do genes do?

 Genes are like a blueprint passed on from parent to child. Proteins are is produced and metabolized according to this genetic blueprint, so we can say that we are kept alive by genetic activities.
Genes have important roles in maintaining our health.
This is why if genes get oxidized by ROS, it can lead to aging and illnesses.

Drinking hydrogen water produces a hormone called ghrelin in the stomach, which protects the cranial nerves. Hydrogen is beneficial to many different organs, from genes to cranial nerves.

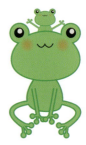

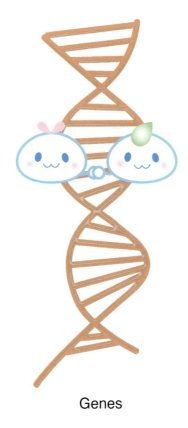

Genes

Promoting Fat Metabolism

 Among the various functions of H_2 is the improvement of our body composition.

 Changing the body to burn more fat.

 The stress caused by oxidation produces a substance called 4-hydroxynonenal (4-HNE), which not only causes "old person smell", but reduces fat metabolism.

 Does that mean that H_2 increases fat metabolism?

 Yes, it does. Genetic functions are complex and there remains much room for further research, but hydrogen has largely two functions: "anti-oxidation" and "genetic health care".
We found out through recent studies how H_2 regulates gene expression by reducing oxidative stress.
We also learned that H_2 modifies inflammatory cytokines, and ROS-produced lipid mediators, which helps explains how hydrogen controls the genetic function.

 And reduces excessive immunity! H_2 is more potent when oxidative stress causes some abnormality within the body.

Hydrogen Reducing Fatigue

 H_2 is most unique compared to existing drugs and medications...

 Because it is also beneficial for perfectly healthy people?

That's right. Normally, when you get sick you go see the doctor, who then examines you and prescribes which drug to take. Each medication corresponds to certain illnesses, but hydrogen deals with the root causes.

Stomachics are only effective for the stomach, but H_2 has effect on the stomach and also for the brain.

Doctors decide who is sick and who is not, but ROS are constantly produced inside our body. For example, by taking hydrogen water we can reduce lactate (lactic acid) build-up, which correlates with not getting as tired after the same amount of workout.

Being tired is not being sick, but H_2 improves the sick and maintains health for those who are not.

Hydrogen does not build up

 H_2 does not stay in one place for long. We must go now, too.

 Because of your dispersing nature, H_2 quickly leaves our body and on its way it reacts with toxic bad ROS. If there are no bad ROS, then it still leaves. That's why it doesn't build up in our body, nor cause side effects.

 Yes! You can consume us without worrying about side effects!

 I believe that hydrogen's wonderful benefits will help many people lead a healthy and joyful life.

 There's sure to be more and more products in the future. We might one day look back with surprise to the days when we didn't consume H_2 on a daily basis.
Thank you Dr. Walter for the great lecture to us hydrogen molecules.
See you again soon!

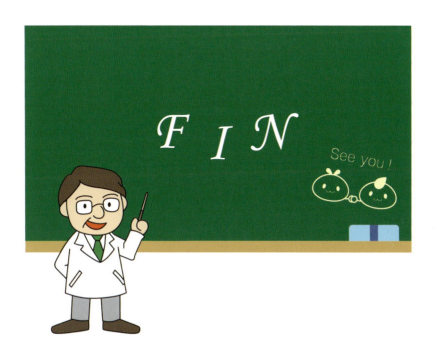

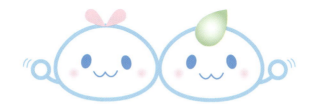

Postscript
by Professor Shigeo Ohta

Molecular hydrogen was believed to be non-functional in our body for a long time. Under this situation, we found that hydrogen exerts important roles for preventive and therapeutic medicine using various disease model animals. The conclusion was obtained as based on standard scientific methods. Now, many clinical studies are underway and most of them have showed positive results. Thus, it is highly expected that hydrogen would be used for general heath care as well as therapy and prevention.

Hydrogen is effective for various kinds of diseases. As far as I know, the effect of hydrogen is greatest. We must think by a different way compared to the conventional drugs and foods.

Although hydrogen is well-known, the efficacy of hydrogen may be too good. This may make people feel skeptical about the great efficacy of hydrogen. Thus, it is important to know the right knowledge on hydrogen.

This small book summarized the properties of hydrogen and the possibility of actual use of hydrogen. If one would read this book, the readers would easily understand the possibility of hydrogen for our heath by deep scientific understandings. This book covers most knowledge about hydrogen. It is very important to distinguish scientific results form pseudoscience.

Hydrogen is **A**pplicable for medical uses without adverse effects, shows **B**road effects as a **C**ompetent molecule with **D**eep scientific understandings and has **E**conomic and Ecologic advantages.

The author is my second son, and I am very proud that he wrote an excellent book about hydrogen.

Shigeo Ohta

Professor, Department of Biochemistry and Cell Biology,
Insitute of Development and Aging Sciences,
Graduate School of Medicine, Nippon Medical School

References

1. Ohsawa I, Ishikawa M, Takahashi K, Watanabe M, Nishimaki K, Yamagata K, Katsura K, Katayama Y, Asoh S, Ohta S. Hydrogen acts as a therapeutic antioxidant by selectively reducing cytotoxic oxygen radicals. *Nat Med*. 2007; 13(6): 688-94. doi: 10.1038/nm1577.

2. Buchholz BM, Kaczorowski DJ, Sugimoto R, Yang R, Wang Y, Billiar TR, McCurry KR, Bauer AJ, Nakao A.: Hydrogen inhalation ameliorates oxidative stress in transplantation induced intestinal graft injury. *Am J Transplant.* 2008; 8(10):2015-24. doi: 10.1111/j.1600-6143.2008.02359.x.

3. Itoh T, Fujita Y, Ito M, Masuda A, Ohno K, Ichihara M, Kojima T, Nozawa Y, Ito M.: Molecular hydrogen suppresses FceRI-mediated signal transduction and prevents degranulation of mast cells. *Biochem Biophys Res Commun*. 2009;389(4):651-6. doi: 10.1016/j.bbrc.2009.09.047.

4. Kamimura N, Nishimaki K, Ohsawa I, Ohta S.: Molecular hydrogen improves obesity and diabetes by inducing hepatic FGF21 and stimulating energy metabolism in db/db mice. *Obesity (Silver Spring)*. 2011;19(7):1396-403. doi: 10.1038/oby.2011.6.

5. Matsumoto A, Yamafuji M, Tachibana T, Nakabeppu Y, Noda M, Nakaya H.: Oral 'hydrogen water' induces neuroprotective ghrelin secretion in mice. *Sci Rep*. 2013;3:3273. doi: 10.1038/srep03273.

6. Iuchi K, Imoto A, Kamimura N, Nishimaki K, Ichimiya H, Yokota T, Ohta S.: Molecular hydrogen regulates gene expression by modifying the free radical chain reaction-dependent generation of oxidized phospholipid mediators. *Sci Rep*. 2016 ;6:18971. doi: 10.1038/srep18971.

7. Aoki K, Nakao A, Adachi T, Matsui Y, Miyakawa S.: Pilot study: Effects of drinking hydrogen-rich water on muscle fatigue caused by acute exercise in eliteathletes. *Med Gas Res.* 2012;2:12. doi: 10.1186/2045-9912-2-12..

8. Kamimura N, Ichimiya H, Iuchi K, Ohta S: Molecular hydrogen stimulates the gene expression of transcriptional c oactivator PGC-1α to enhance fatty acid metabolism. *npj Aging and Mechanisms of Disease 2*: 2016;16008. doi:10.1038/npjamd.2016.8

9. Simon AR: Hydrogen-supplemented drinking water, just soda or an elixir of life? *Transpl Int.* 2012;25(12):1211-2. doi: 10.1111/j.1432-2277.2012.01574.x.

10. Ichihara M, Sobue S, Ito M, Ito M, Hirayama M, Ohno K.: Beneficial biological effects and the underlying mechanisms of molecular hydrogen - comprehensive review of 321 original articles. *Med Gas Res*. 2015;5:12. doi: 10.1186/s13618-015-0035-1.

11. Nicolson GL, Mattos GF, Settineri R, Costa C, Ellithorpe R, Rosenblatt S, Valle JL, Jimenez A, Ohta S.: Clinical Effects of Hydrogen Administration: From Animal and Human Diseases to Exercise Medicine. *Int J Clin Med* 2016; 7:32-76. doi.org/10.4236/ijcm.2016.71005.

Special Thanks
to
Shigeo Ohta, Ph.D.

Illustrator
Momoko Sakaguchi
A.I
Noriko Kitabatake
SATSUKI

Translator
Rina Otani
Reiko Kameda

Proofreader
Tyler W. LeBaron
(Molecular Hydrogen Foundation)

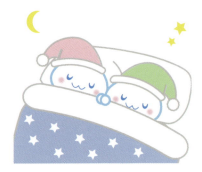

【著者紹介】

おおたふみあき（Fumiaki Ohta）

1981年、福島県生まれ。
水素の医学、健康、美容分野への応用の研究開発を行う。
著書に『ウォルター先生の水素のはなし』（産学社）。

【監修と解説】

太田成男（Shigeo Ohta）

日本医科大学大学院医学研究科細胞生物学分野　大学院教授。
1951年、福島県生まれ。1974年、東京大学理学部卒業。
1979年、東京大学大学院薬学系研究科博士課程を修了した後、
スイス・バーゼル大学バイオセンター研究所研究員、
自治医科大学講師・助教授を経て、1994年より現職。
30年以上に及ぶ研究から、ミトコンドリアに備わっている機能が
心身の健康と密接に関わり、水素の抗酸化作用が有効であることを発見する。
日本ミトコンドリア学会前理事長（現理事）、日本Cell Death学会前理事長（現評議員）、
分子状水素医学生物学会理事長などを務めている。
『体が若くなる技術』(サンマーク出版)、
瀬名秀明との共著『ミトコンドリアと生きる』(角川書店)、
瀬名秀明との共著『ミトコンドリアのちから』(新潮社)、
『水素水とサビない身体』(小学館)、
安保徹との共著『老いない人の健康術』(産学社) など著書多数。

Professor. Shigeo Ohta ,Nippon Medical School.
1951 was born.
1974 was graduated from the University of Tokyo.
1979 Received phD.
1981 Research on Mitochondrial Biogenesis.
1985 Mitochondrial Disease.
1994 Oxidative stress from mitochondria.
2005 Hydrogen Medicine.

These profile of first edition remain on the revised one.

HYDROGEN

初版 1刷発行 ●2016年　9月15日
2版 2刷発行 ●2019年 10月10日

著　者
おおたふみあき

発行者
薗部 良徳

発行所
㈱産学社

〒101-0061 東京都千代田区神田三崎町2-20-7 水道橋西口会館
Tel.03（6272）9313　Fax.03（3515）3660
http://www.sangakusha.jp/

印刷所
㈱ティーケー出版印刷

©Fumiaki Ohta 2016, Printed in Japan
ISBN978-4-7825-3459-5 C2076

乱丁、落丁本はお手数ですが当社営業部宛にお送りください。
送料当社負担にてお取り替えいたします。
本書の内容の一部または全部を無断で複製、掲載、転載することを禁じます。